The Complete Guide to Pharmacy: A Comprehensive Handbook

Dr Raafet

Published by Dr Raafet, 2023.

THE COMPLETE GUIDE TO PHARMACY: A COMPREHENSIVE HANDBOOK

First edition. July 16, 2023.

ISBN: 979-8223618096

Written by Dr Raafet.

Summary

Pharmacy

I. Legal framework

Legal definition of a pharmacy

"Retail pharmacy means the establishment assigned to the filling of magistral prescriptions, to the preparation of medicinal products listed in the pharmacopoeia defined in Article 28 of this Law and to the retail sale of the products referred to in Article 21 of this Law."

Article 10 of Law 73-55 of 3 August 1973:

Distribution of pharmacies in Tunisia:

Two categories:

Category A pharmacies: pharmacie by day

Category B pharmacies: night pharmacy

Condition for the creation of a pharmacy:

The operation of a pharmacy requires obtaining an operating license

this is awarded by order of the Minister of Public Health (MSP) after advice from CNOP, the order must mention the category of license (A or B).

The conditions are:

› Be of Tunisian nationality for 5 years.
› Be equipped with a degree of doctoreur in pharmacy.
› Be in good standing with the law for military service (male)
Ø Be registered with the Order of Pharmacists .
› Have a blameless criminal record.

The opening and closing hours of the pharmacy:

The opening and closing hours of category A retail pharmacies are fixed, for the days of the week, by an order of the MSP

	1ers e ptembreto31Mai		1erj u inau31Augustut	
	Opening	*Closure*	*Opening*	*Closure*
Morning	08:30	13:00	08:00	1:30 pm
Afternoon	15:00	7:30 pm	16:00	20:00
Saturday	08:30	13:00	08:00	1:30 pm

Organization of the Guards:

Childcare is organized to meet the needs of the public outside of business hours

It is insured:

	1ers e ptembreto31Mai		1erj u inau31Augustut	
From Saturday to Friday, the days	***Opening***	***Closure***	***Opening***	***Closure***
Holidays	08:30	7:30 pm	08:00	20:00

The distribution of guards is done according to a schedule that takes into consideration separately:

- National holidays
- Religious holidays
- Ordinary days

Pharmacies are informed of their on-call duties by means of a guard board at the beginning of each year. The Regional Council of Order of Pharmacists divided the category A pharmacies of a region into lists. The pharmacies belonging to the same list simultaneously provide guard in order to cover the whole city.

Each pharmacy is obliged to post the list of on-call pharmacies outside the pharmacy in a place visible to patients

The standards required for a pharmacy

- Article 1: any premises intended for the establishment of a retail pharmacy must include:

- A sales room intended for the public, whose ceiling height must be at least two meters eighty centimeters (2m 80).

- A drop-off room and a laboratory (must be sufficiently ventilated)

- A toilet

- A pharmacist's office

◈ Article 2:The total useful surface area required for the approval of the premises must be at least fifty square metres (50 m2) of which at least thirty metres (30 m2) must be on the ground.

◈ Article 3: The technical equipment of the pharmacy premises must include the material and facilities necessary for the proper functioning of the pharmacy, in particular running water, electricity, telephone and refrigerator.

◈ Article 4: Any premises intended for the creation of a retail pharmacy must first be approved by the Ministry of Public Health after consulting the Council of the Order of Pharmacists.

II. Layout of the pharmacy

Auction room:

The sales room is reserved to welcome patients and serve them efficiently and confidentially. It must be spacious and welcoming, furnished with maximum order and cleanliness.

The auction room generally has two areas separated by the counter:

› An area accessible to patients where dermo-cosmetic products, hygiene products and baby accessories stored in displays are displayed

› An area not accessible to patients, located behind the counter, with shelves containing products advice of wide rotation, dietary products, food supplements .... As well as a cabinet with sliding drawers where the pharmaceutical specialties are stored and classified by form and alphabetical order.

› The counter where the computers are arranged with a box underneath, a barcode reader, office accessories (pens, corrector, scissors, stapler ...)

Drop-off room:

It is accessible to staff only. It contains shelves containing all pharmaceutical products in stock. There is also a refrigerator for temperature-sensitive products whose conservation is between +2 ° C and + 8 ° C

Injection room:

It is a space that preserves the privacy of the patient. There is all the necessary equipment for the practice of injections: syringes, antiseptic solutions, compresses, cotton, a garbage can.

The laboratory:

It is a very equipped space, where magistral and officinal preparations are carried out. It is perfectly clean, equipped with a bench, electricity, running water and a heat source.

It contains the raw material used to ensure the preparations, the necessary preparation material, the register of compendial preparations where the name of the preparation, the quantity prepared and the date of the preparation are mentioned.

Pharmacist's Office:

In his office, the pharmacist manages the pharmacy and sometimes receives representatives and delegates of pharmaceutical and parapharmaceutical laboratories.

The office is equipped with a telephone, a computer linked to the local network, a library with scientific books (Vidal, the therapeutic form, the preparer's manual, the pharmacopoeia,...) and a locked cabinet reserved for narcotics.

Management of the pharmacy

I. Stock management

The pharmacist must be able to establish a state of equilibriumbetweeninputsand outputsand betweenoverstockand stock-outs. Thismakes it possible to avoid expenditure due to storage and expired products. Thus, a good officinal ensures and controls the application of the following rules:

- Adapt purchases to the needs of the patient, the epidemiological context and the season
- Avoid over-stocking of low-turnover products
- Refuse products on close dates upon receipt of orders
- Consider expiration dates when selling using the First In First Out (FIFO) rule

1. Fulfilment of orders

The order is the first step in the supply of medicines, it is carried out by the pharmacist or the preparers.

To optimize the management of his business, the pharmacist must control his stock so as not to have

› On storage: immobilization of money but also a loss (increased risk of having expired products)

› Understocking: risk of out of stock or missed sales

The right balance must be found to optimize stock management. For this, the pharmacist takes into account certain criteria when preparing an order:

- Product exit movements (rotational speed)

- Quantities in stock

- Storage capacity

- The value of the stock

- The expiry date

- The seasonality of certain medications.

- Promotions

Orders are made with suppliers or wholesale distributors.

The choice of suppliers must be established according to specific criteria including:

› The proximity between the pharmacy and the depot (speed of delivery).

› The importance of the wholesaler distributor in stock volume (availability of products).

› The conditions of payment (delivery or instalments of drafts).

› The quality of service offered

Types of commands:

1. Daily order:

Performed on a daily basis to keep a minimum amount of stock. The order is placed by telephone with the nearest suppliers.

This type of order is made on average 2 to 4 times a day.

Orders placed in the morning or afternoon arrive the same day and those ordered in the evening arrive the next morning

2. Group order:

Concerns products with high turnover and whose consumption is almost linear throughout the year and whose expiry date does not pose problems.

Example: analgesics, anti-inflammatory ....

This order depends on storage capacity, financial status and the existence of a promotional sale. It aims to lighten daily orders and/or to prepare for a guard.

3. Urgent order:

These are orders made for products that must be delivered within the same hour; They are carried out with wholesalers close geographically.

They concern products not available at the pharmacy level or when the quantity present is insufficient.

The steps of realization of an order:

1. Order preparation:

is made according to the type of order, we note in an order book, the specialties, pharmaceutical products and parapharmaceutical articles to order from wholesalers distributors by telephone.

2. Receipt of an order:

At each reception, we must check:

› the name of the pharmacist on the packaging

› The supplier's name, address and contact details

› The presence of a delivery note (BL).

› The conformity of the quantities received with those mentioned on the delivery note.

› The integrity of the container and contents.

› Presence of vignettes (products with vignettes).

› Expiry dates (close dates< 6 months will be returned to the supplier)

› Respect for the cold chain for temperature-sensitive products (the first to be treated).

› The characteristics of each product: its PCT code, its description, the quantity delivered, the unit price excluding tax and the public selling price

› To the selling price is added the pharmacist's liability fee which is:

+ 240 millimes for the specialities of Tables A and C

+ 300 millimes for the specialities in Table B

› Any price changes must be corrected in the corresponding article sheet

In case of non-conformity (receipt of an erroneous product, not ordered or received by excess or default, having an expiry date close or already expired) the products are returned as soon as possible to the supplier and it is necessary to make a claim to the supplier within a period not exceeding 48 hours which, in return will send a voucher.

3. Computer entry

› Entering the name of the supplier

› Order form number

› Date of order

› Entry of items and quantities received

› Verification if the amount obtained corresponds to that of the invoice

In case of non-compliance, the purchase price of each product is checked

In the case of a new product, we must then create the product sheet that includes:

- Description of the drug (bar code, trade name, table, category, form)

- Scientific parameters (active ingredient, indications

- specific)

- Sales parameters (PAHT, VAT, PTTC)

- The parameters of the CNAM (PCT code, refunded or not...)

After validation, note "registered" on the BL and store it in a folder containing all the BLs of the current month of the supplier in question.

4. The establishment:

Medications are stored while making sure to rank those with the earliest expiry date first to be sold first.

The proper storage of medications is an essential factor in ensuring an excellent quality of service in terms of safety and speed

2. Monthly invoice scoring

Each supplier sends a summary of the previous month's purchases in 1 copy at the beginning of the month. One remains with the pharmacist and the other is returned to the supplier after verification. Invoices can be paid:

- By cheque
- By bank transfer
- Partraite

3. Inventory

❖ It is carried out in order to correct discrepancies between the theoretical stock displayed by the computer system and the physical stock.

The interest of the inventory is the adjustment of the stock. It is also a means of warning to make the necessary returns of the dates of close expiry.

❖ There are severaltypes of inventory:

Daily inventory: made daily upon receipt of the order and targets the products ordered

Annual inventory: It is mandatory to know the value of the stock at the end of the year in order to communicate it to the accountant for the purposes of the annual balance sheet. It is a globalinventoryofall the medicines and articles existing in the pharmacy.

4. Management of expired products

❖ Expired products are a major problem because of the financial damage they cause. So to minimize as much as possible the generation of expired ones, the pharmacist and his preparers must:

• Avoid overstock

• Store medications so that the nearest date is always placed in front. In this way, expiry dates are regularly checked.

• Refuse products with a close expiry date at the order level, especially for products with low turnover

• Continuously control the expiry date of each product and mark the products at close date

❖ Once the products have expired, they are immediately removed from the shelves, stored in sports cartons visibly marked 'expired' and held in the pharmacy in a place reserved for them in such a way as to avoid confusion with the stock of medicinal products.

❖ These products will be noted on a list and subsequently destroyed in the presence of a bailiff and a member of the regional tax directorate.

This list will be sent to the Ministry of Finance for the tax exemption and to the Ministry of the Environment for the destruction authorization.

II. Financial Management

The pharmacist belongs to the real regime, i.e. he/she is required to have accounting with an accountant and financial statements. Before opening his pharmacy, the pharmacist must apply for registration in the commercial regime in order to have a licence

1. Social obligations

❖ The pharmacist must join the CNSS as an employer and as a staff. He must also join his employees and pay the contributions set by the CNSS

.

❖ It must comply with the Labour Code and the collective agreements between the pharmacists' union and the pharmacy employees' union.

2. Commercial obligations

The pharmacist must register in the commercial register and keep complete and updated accounts.

3. Tax obligations

Monthly declaration :

12 declarations / year
Before the 15th of each month, the pharmacist must file the tax return for the previous month.

Quarterly Statement

Declaration to the National Social Security Fund (CNSS):
This declaration includes the monthly salary and the total salaries. It is drawn up in 3 copies,one remains at the pharmacy,the other two are

sent to the CNSS.The pharmacist must pay 2 contributions on the gross quarterly salary:

- A contribution of 25.75% (social contribution)
- A contribution of 0.5% (contribution for accidents at work)

Annual declaration: single declaration of income (DUR)

Before April 25 of each year, the pharmacist must present to the tax authorities a document that closes his annual turnover, the instalment and what remains to be paid.

If the statement has been advanced to the amount greater than the annual profit, a rebound is requested that will be withdrawn from next year's instalments.

Instalment payments:

It is an advance to the state of 30% of the amount of the single declaration of income paid the previous year.

It is done on 3 tranches

Employer's Statement:

This is a statement of the entire list of employees of the whole year with their total salary

III. Human resources management

Human resources management is one of the fundamental axes of successful pharmacy management. The community pharmacist must:

› Define the needs of his establishment in personnel and the associated skills.

› Manage recruitment, integration and training of staff.

› Regularly evaluate the skills of its employees.

› Distribute and plan activities according to constraints (absences ....).

› Create an operational body specifying the role of each employee.

› Develop a control device

The employer-employee relationship is governed by regulations'

› The labour code that applies to all employees

› Collective agreements that complement the Labour Code and normalize the pharmacist's relationship with his employer

› These agreements improve the status of employees and organize the rules specific to the sector of activity, the probationary period, hygiene, safety, the different levels of the employee.

Staff recruitment:

Different recruitment methods are used

› Employees can be recruited through the employment office.

› Trainee preparers who have completed their end-of-study internship at a pharmacy level may subsequently be recruited by the pharmacist training supervisor if they prove to be sufficiently competent and if the work requires new recruitment.

› To apply for the position of a pharmacist, employees can submit their application to the National Council of the Order of Pharmacists of Tunisia.

The different types of contracts:

ü SIVP: introductory course to professional life:

It is a contract between the employer and the employment office. The employee receives a salary from the employer and one from the state.

The duration of this contract is 1 year non-renewable, the employer in this case is exempt from payment of the CNSS and income tax.

ü CEF: employment training contract:

Concerns preparers and assistant preparers who have not obtained the bachelor's degree.

It is a contract between the pharmacist and his apprentices and is renewable until the end of the training.

ü CDD: fixed-term contract:

It is a trial contract and the employer alone will have the ability to judge the competence of the employee and make the decision to re-recruit him or not.

ü Permanent contract: contract of indefinite duration:

Except in cases of serious misconduct, this may terminate the contract

Establishment of a pay slip:

A pay slip (or pay slip) is drawn up in 2 copies: One copy for the employee and another for the employer. This form must contain the following information:

› The name of the pharmacist and his address.

› The surname/first name of the employee, his CIN number, his CNSS number, his quality, his category, his step.

› The basic salary: this is the salary granted on the basis of the legal number of working hours per month set at 173 hours / month by the collective agreement.

› The number of overtime hours.

› Premiums: cash, transport, presence.

› The CNSS contribution.

› Withholding (tax)

› The gross salary: this is the basic salary plus bonuses and overtime pay.

› The net salary: this is the amount received by the employee after deduction of the CNSS contribution and the deduction of taxes from the gross salary

The certificate of work:

A certificate of work is a document written by the pharmacist at the request of the employee, it mentions:

› Surname/first name and address of pharmacist.

› Surname/first name, ID number and status of the employee.

› Pharmacist's signature and stamp

Paid leave:

Every employee is entitled to one month of paid leave per year, in addition to public holidays and religious holidays

Other paid leave:

› Maternity leave: duration = 2 months.

› Sick leave: The employee must provide a medical certificate within 48 hours, he can then benefit from 5 days of paid leave, beyond these 5 days it is the CNSS that takes care of him

Working hours

Each employee will work 40 hours / week or 173 hours / month.

Overtime:

› The first 32 hours we have an increase of 25%.

› Beyond that we have an increase of 50%.

For a breastfeeding woman the number of hours / week is reduced to 34 hours / week for (1 hour of feeding / day), this is valid for a period of 6 months.

Medicinal product

I. Definition of medicinal product

According to article 21 of law 73-55 organizing the pharmaceutical professions:

'A medicinal product shall mean any substance or combination of substances presented for treating and preventing disease in humans or animals and any product which may be administered to humans or animals with a view to making a medical diagnosis or restoring, correcting or modifying their organic functions.'

II. Classification and storage of medicinal products

Medications are arranged in a precise order

> In alphabetical order

> by dosage form

> The storage of the same medication is done according to the expiry date

> Table B products and psychotropic drugs are stored in a locked cabinet in the pharmacist's office

> Homeopathic and phytotherapeutic medicines Dermocosmetic products and parapharmaceutical products are stored in separate shelves so that they are clearly visible to the public

1. Proprietary medicinal products

Medicines are arranged at:

❖ Shelvesbehindthecounter:They are easily accessible to the pharmacist.

We have 4 compartments, each consisting of several shelves

- 1st compartment: there are the consulting products
- 2nd compartment: there is the Formesirop
- 3rd compartment: homeopathic medicines
- 4th compartment: there are nasal forms

❖ Sliding drawers: they allow the storage of other pharmaceuticalforms

› Tablets and capsules
› Mouthwashes
› Eye drops and ophthalmic ointment
› Sachets
› Etovule suppositories
› Lesointments
› Injectable forms
› Drinkable drops
› Solutions for external use

2. Infant formula

The milks are organized in a display (not exposed to the public) classified according to age or a special indication.

A distinction is made between milks of:

› 1st age: from 0 to 6 months
› 2nd age: from 6 months to 1 year
› 3rd age: from 1 to 3 years old

There are also milks with special properties such as:

› ☹◈◈⧫□◈◈◈◈▫◈◈ milks (LF): PRIMALAC LF (LactoseFree)

> Anti-colic milks (AC): PRIMALAC digest AC, MODILACAC
> Anti-constipation milks (CS)

3. Parapharmaceutical products

They include:

◈ Dermo-cosmetic products: they are distributed according to the mode of use, the indication and the manufacturer laboratory (Avene®, SVR® ...) in shelves accessible to customers. • Food supplements: they are visible to customers and more easily accessible to staff than conventional medicines.

◈ Food supplements: they are visible to customers and more easily accessible to staff than conventional drugs.

III. Legislation and management relating to products belonging to different productstables

Reminders:

❖ Poisonous substances are classified in 3 tables:

- Table C or List II: dangerous products.
- Table A or List I: toxic substances
- Table B: narcotic drugs

❖ If the poisonous raw material is found in the medicinal product at a dose less than or equal to that indicated in the exemption tables, the medicinal product is exempt and is not included in the corresponding category.

1. The products in Table A and C

Table A: "Toxic products": They have a strong intrinsic toxicity even at very low dosages. They can cause serious toxic effects. Their administration requests medical surveillance

Table C: "Hazardous Products": They have a lower intrinsic toxicity. Their administration can accommodate less close medical surveillance. Risks of serious toxic effects are lower

(a) Labelling

Tableau A	Tableau C
Voies internes : orale, perlinguale, rectale, vaginale, urétrale ou transcutanée + Contre étiquette RESPECTER LES DOSES PRESCRITES	
Voies externes : nasales, oculaires, auriculaires, collutoire, gargarisme et cutanée + Contre étiquette RESPECTER LES DOSES PRESCRITES NE PAS AVALER	

(b) Detention

These products are kept out of the reach of patients in shelves with sliding drawers or they are classified by dosage form and alphabetically.

(c) Dispensation

The dispensing of these products is done only on medical prescription. The order is returned to the patient after having:

- Transcribed the price and date of dispensing
- Mentioned the transcription number to the authorising officer and the quantity issued
- Affixed the stamp

(d) Renewal

Table A: Medicinal products containing substances in Table A, with the exception of those intended to be applied to the skin, may be renewed only when the prescriber is in writing and after the period determined by the instructions for use indicated in the prescription.

Table C: The prescription is renewable, unless otherwise advised by the prescriber and after the period determined by the instructions for use.

2. Special cases of certain psychotropic substances

(a) Definition

Psychotropic drugs are drugs that alter mental activity. Some psychotropic drugs are subject to special legislation (circulars) because of their high toxicity and increased risk of dependence:

› Trihexyphenidyl (PARKIZOL®5mg tablet B/50)
› Clonazepam(CLONAZEPAM®2mg scored tabletB/40)
› Diazepam (VALIUM®10mg scored tablet B/30)
› Lorazepam (TEMESTA 2.5mg B/30 and TEMESTA®®1mg B/30)

(b) Supply

The supply of these products is made by a specific order form signed by the pharmacist in person which is mentioned:

- Name and surname of pharmacist
- The address of the pharmacy.
- date.
- Quantities in full of the products ordered and delivered.
- Signature and stamp of the pharmacist and the supplier.
- The strains signed by the supplier are kept by the pharmacist.

(c) Detention

Storage takes place out of the reach of persons outside the establishment and specially reserved for these products. As a precaution, they can be kept in a lockable cabinet in the pharmacist's office.

(d) Dispensation

❖ Dispensing is carried out exclusively by the community pharmacist installed in the governorate of the place of practice of the doctor, prescribed: the patient's residence.

❖ These medicinal products should only be issued on a blue medical prescription, numbered and taken from a stock booklet, distributed by the National Council of the Order of Doctors of Tunisia. The patient's national identity card or third party is required.The order must include:

○ Surname, first name, address, telephone number and stamp of the prescribing physician

○ Surname, first name, CIN and address of the patient

○ Name of the drug, dosage, dosage form, dosage and duration of treatment which should not exceed 90 days.

❖ In the execution of the order, the following must be checked:

› The absence of the association ClonazepametTrihexyphenidyl and unless otherwise stated "I do say "

› The absence of overlaps, excessive dosages and automatic renewals of treatments.

› The pharmacist keeps only a copy of the prescribed prescription

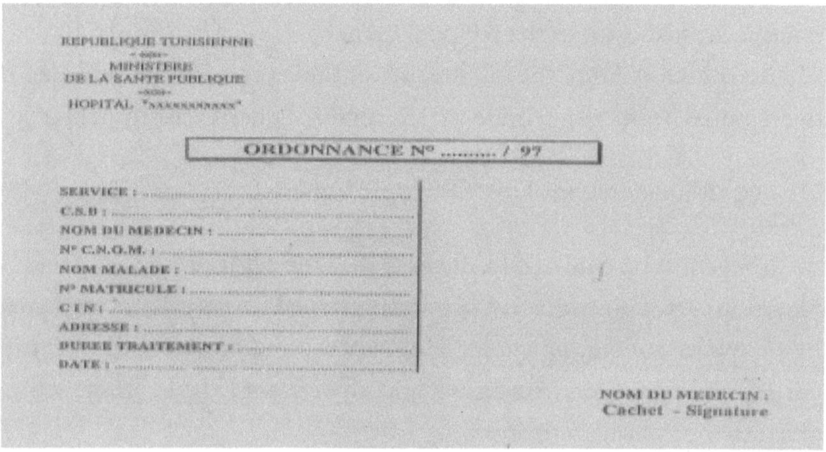
REPUBLIQUE TUNISIENNE

MINISTERE
DE LA SANTE PUBLIQUE

HOPITAL "xxxxxxxxxx"

ORDONNANCE N° .... / 97

SERVICE :
C.S.B :
NOM DU MEDECIN :
N° C.N.O.M. :
NOM MALADE :
N° MATRICULE :
C I N :
ADRESSE :
DUREE TRAITEMENT :
DATE :

NOM DU MEDECIN :
Cachet - Signature

(e) Transcript on authorising officer

It shall be made in GREEN ink, the particulars to be entered in the authorising officer are:

- The date of execution of the order.
- The name of the prescribing physician.
- The serial number.
- The galenic form.
- The name of the medicine.
- The quantity delivered
- The name and surname of the patient.
- The national identity card number (CIN)

The pharmacist must write on the prescription the transcription number on the authorizing officer of each product dispensed to the patient, the date, the stamp of the pharmacy and his signature

(f) Management of psychotropic drugs

A quarterly sales report after the end of each quarter is sent to the pharmacist inspector of the regional branch.

After each quarter, the sales report of these products is forwarded to the regional health directorate (to the regional pharmacist inspector).

(g) Management of psychotropic hopeds

They must be removed from the real, computerized stock and will be placed in boxes on which its 'psychotrophoped' written is accompanied by an invoice containing a complete list of expired products, the quantity corresponding to each speciality and their expiry dates. They will be given to the pharmacistinspector.

3. Narcotics

(a) Definition

Schedule B products or narcotics are addictive and consequently progressively degrade the psychic, somatic and social capacities of the individual.

(b) Labelling

Double red frame with a counter label "Respect the prescribed doses".

(c) Procurement

❖ Procurement requires a pink order form extracted from a stump booklet. These instalence booklets are distributed by the CNOPT and are rated and initialled by the regional pharmacist inspector. The purchase order has three parts: 1 stump component and 2 acquit-à-caution parts. The voucher must be written in ink, legible, without erasures or overloads.

❖ The strain mentions:

• Surname, first name and address of the pharmacist

• Names of the products requested and quantities in full

• Name of supplier

• Dates, signature, etc. of the pharmacist owner of the pharmacy.

› The other two panes contain the same information and are sent to the supplier. Then the supplier returns one of the shutters to the pharmacist after having affixed his stamp and signature indicating the exit number in his register, the date of delivery and the quantity delivered (in words).

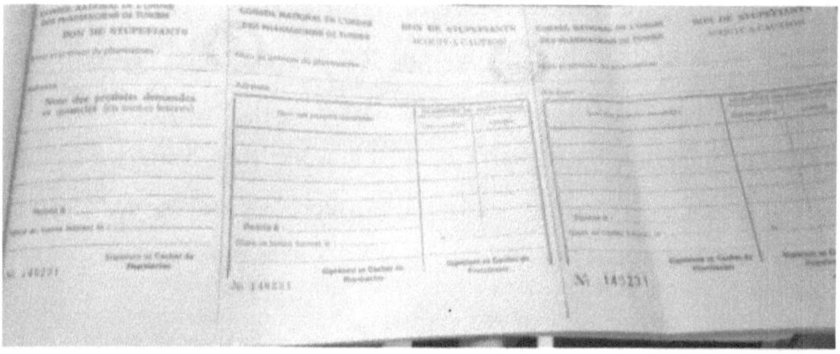

› The shelf life of the stumps and flaps is 10 years from 31 December of the current year.

(d) Detention

Schedule B medications are kept in the pharmacist's office in a locked double-turn safe. The keys must be held by the pharmacist himself.

(e) Dispensation

◈ 3 Mandatory conditions to check

› A prescription for Schedule B products is dispensed by a retail pharmacist in the governorate of the prescription in the governorate where the patient's place of residence is **located (geographical limitation)**

› This order may not be carried out after forty-eight hours(48) of the day it is issued. If the prescription is submitted after the aforementioned period, it can only be filled for the remainder of the treatment period in accordance with what is prescribed on the prescription **(validity period)**

› It is prohibited to prescribe and dispensing Schedule B substances in oral or transdermal form for a period exceeding 28 days. For Schedule B substances in injectable form, this period cannot exceed 14 days **(duration of treatment)**

❖ The prescription is extracted from a booklet printed by the Council of the Order of Physicians or Dentists. The order must include the following information:

- Surname, first name, address, telephone number and stamp of the prescribing doctor

- Surname, first name and address of the patient

• Serial number of the instanticil booklet

• Date of prescription in full

• Designation of the product with dosage and dosage form, dosage and duration of treatment mentioned in full.

(f) Transcript on the authorising officer

❖ It shall be carried out at the RED INK mentioning:

• The date of issue

• The name of the prescriber and his/her address

• The transcription number to the authorising officer

• The name and dosage form of the medicinal product, the quantity dispensed in full

• The name and address of the patient or of the third person responsible for obtaining the treatment, together with the national identity card number.

❖ After transcription on the authorising officer, the pharmacist must write on the prescription: the registration number to the authorising officer, the date of dispensing, the quantity delivered, the stamp of the pharmacy and the price of the medicinal product

These prescriptions must be kept with the pharmacist for 10 years after December 31 of the dispensing year

(a) Desperate management

❖ Obsolete Table B products are kept by the pharmacist until the visit of the pharmacist inspector (he is the only one authorized to destroy them). The pharmacist inspector therefore proceeds to count and destroy them (the tablets will be crushed and thrown away, the injectables broken and then crushed empty) and notes on the register of entries and exits at the level of the part reserved for the monthly exits of the destroyed products, the quantities destroyed and the new stock in full by affixing his stamp, his signature and the date of his visit.

❖ In the event of fortuned destruction of a morphine ampoule, a notary bailiff must be called in to draw up a report to show it to the regional inspector pharmacist.

Pharmacy advice

Pharmacy advice:

The pharmacist is very much in demand for pharmacy advice, whether it is medication advice or hygiene advice, for the following reasons:

› The pharmacist is competent (long studies). He knows the drug, its indications and its side effects

› Access to advice by the patient is very easy and free unlike the medical consultation where you have to make an appointment and pay the costs of a consultation. This does not mean that the pharmacist can replace the doctor but that pharmacy advice is very important to master. Advice does not necessarily mean giving a medicine

Reception of a patient seeking advice:

› Confidentiality: The dialogue between the pharmacist and the patient must be established in a confidential area, thus creating a climate of trust facilitating the interrogation

› Interrogation aims to assess the severity of symptoms and verify that there is no interference with ongoing treatment or self-medication or with the patient's medical condition

› Know how to refer to the doctor

› Avoid medical procedures

Study of consulting cases

Headaches

The interrogation plays a very important role in knowing the exact causes of the pain, its etiology, its type and intensity as well as the circumstances of its appearance.

› Paracetamol (per os): Efferalgan, Doliprane®, , Panadol®, Analgan®®, ...

The dosage should not exceed 4g / d with an intake every 6 hours (less if there are liver problems) and 60mg / kg / day for children.

› Acetyl salicylic acid (ASA): Aspirin tablet ®Aspégic1000®

Note: The pharmacological properties of ASA are dose dependent.

Dosage	Pharmacological property (in adults)
>4g	Uricosuric action
>3g/day	Anti-inflammatory action
1 to 3 g/day	Antipyretic and analgesic action
<1g	Antiplatelet agent Example: Kardegic ® 160 mg (lysine acetylsalicylate) for the treatment of acute MI

The sore throat

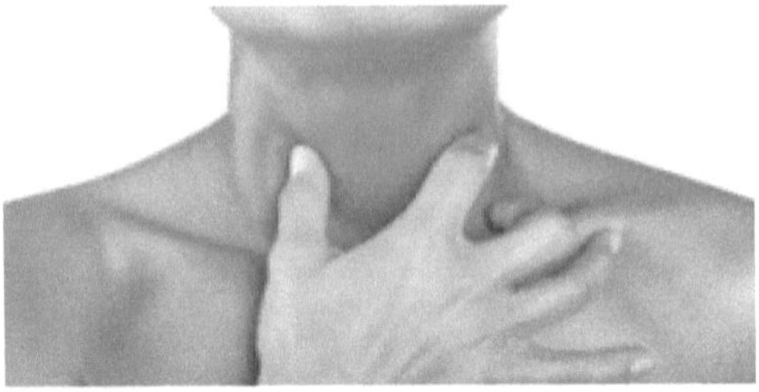

❖ **Description:**

The sore throat is often accompanied by inflammation. It may be diffuse or localised to the tonsils, pharynx or aularynx.

❖ **Classic symptoms:**

◈ Tingling, difficulty swallowing solid food. Bad breath, hoarseness of the throat.

◈ It is mainly through interrogation that the disgorge is recognised, and the pharmacist is not entitled to observe the shape and tonsilla colour.

❖ **Treatment:**

ü An antiseptic for disinfection: Verax blu®, Hexaspray®

ü An analgesic based on paracetamol: Doliprane®, Panadol®, Algeci®, Efferalgan vitC®

ü Drill® lozenges to suck (honey, sugar-free, lemon mint): This medication contains an antiseptic (Chlorhexidine) which has an antibacterial effect and a local anesthetic effect (Tetracaine) which is analgesic.

ü An anti-inflammatory:Maxilase®

ü Homeopathic treatment: Homeovox®

❖ **Advice:**

› It is advisable to drink water, prefer hot drinks with honey and lemon.

› Prefer foods in liquid form to reduce swallowing pain

› Throat sowings, hypersalivation caused by sucking contributes to healing.

› Avoid sudden changes in temperature

› Treatment time should not exceed 5 days

Cough

❖ **Description:**

It is a deliberate act orreflexele more often noisy, the aim of which is to remove from the respiratory tree the foreign bodies or secretions that clutter it.

❖ **Classification:**

ü *Dry cough*: causes: cold, pharyngitis, laryngitis, medications(IEC.)

ü *Coughing*:followed by sputum (expulsion of bulky matter)

❖ **Interrogation:**

The interrogation is necessary to define the nature of the cough, the questions to ask:

❖ Is your cough recent?

› If > 3 weeks: chronic cough refer to the doctor

› If < 3 weeks: acute cough

❖ Do you have mucus that forces you to spit?

› Yes: wet cough

› No: dry cough

❖ Is coughing more common morning or evening?

› Morning sputum: smoking cough

› Evening cough: directs us to an allergic cough

❖ Do you have any associated signs (weight loss, headache, chest pain) or hemoptysis?

› Yes: cough can be a symptom of a serious illness referred to the doctor.

❖ Do you have ongoing treatment (ACE)?

› Yes: iatrogenic cough refer to the doctor

❖ **Treatment:**

❖ *Dry cough: Latoux sedatives*

› **Syrups:**

◈ Calmatux® (codeine)

◈ Pecto6® adult (codeine + codetyline) / child (codeine) / infant (sodium benzoate + sodium bromide + thicolor)

◈ Tussipax® Child / Adult (dextrometorphan)

◈ Drill® dry cough (dextrometorphan)

❖ *Wet cough: Bronchial thinners, expectorants, mucolytics, mucoregulators:*

› **Syrups:**

- ® adult/child (carbocistein); Bronchokod® without sugar
- Bronchothiol® adult/child (carbocisteine)
- Rhinathiol® adult/child (carbocisteine)
- Drill expectorant® (carbocisteine)
- Sugar-free Muxol® (Ambroxol); Strong Muxol ®)
- Mucosol® adult/child (carbocisteine)
- Mucolyte® (bromhexine)
- Toplexil® (Guaifenisin +Oxomemazine)

❖ **Associated advice:**

- If the cough is chronic or associated with fever or other signs of complications, refer the patient to the doctor
- Avoid opioids in pregnant and lactating women.
- Use sugar-free syrups in diabetics
- Codeine-based syrups are table specialties
- For children we usually recommend a herbal syrup for example toumix®

Digestive illnesses

1. Diarrhoea

❖ Description

It is defined by the emission of more than 3stool per day and/ or too much liquid for more than 2 days.

It can be viral or bacterial (most often).

❖ Advice to the patient

Dietplays a major roleitisimportantto avoid certain foods (spices,...) which cause irritation and favorite to a diet that gives consistency to sits, such as rice, bananas, yoghurt, etc.

Hydration is an essential factor in case of diarrhea to avoid possible dehydration.

❖ Treatment

- Adsorbents: **Smecta®**...

- Anti-diarrheal substances of microbial origin: **Enterogermminasusp®Ultrayeast®**

- In case of diarrhea accompanied by abdominal spasms: **Spasmocalm® Actafon®**

- Rehydration in infants and children: **Fanolyte®**

❖ **Note**: The patient should be referred to the physician if: diarrhea persists for more than 3 days, presence of fever, weakened or vomiting significant. :

2.Constipation:

❖ Description

In a healthy subject, constipation is called constipation if there is:

- <3stoolper week or<35gdesellesper day(in adults)
- <1saddle/2day(in children)
- <1 bowel movement/day (in infants)

It is necessary to know the character of constipation (recent or old), look for an iatrogenic or drug cause.

❖ Advice to the patient

- Avoid slowing down foods (e.g. rice, choice, bananas, cabbage)

- Drink enoughwater(especially a large glass of water in the morning)

- Favor foods rich in fiber such as green vegetables, certain fruits (apple, grape), olive oil ...

- Practicing physical activity promotes intestinal transit.

❖ Treatment

• Ballast laxatives: **Normacol®** sterculiasachet gum.

• Laxativeslubricants: **Laxafine®syrup.**

• Osmotic laxatives: **Osmolax®, Duphalac®**

• Rectal laxatives:

ü Glycerin-based suppositories:**Glyss® adult**

ü Enemas :**Laxagel® enemas.**

Patient Education

I. Introduction:

Health education is an ethical obligation for pharmacists. The latter must contribute to informing the public about health as the closest and most accessible professional to ducitoyen.

II. Role of the pharmacist:

As part of the therapeutic education of the patient, the pharmacist must:

1. Promote the proper use of the medicine:

When dispensing, the pharmacist must:

• Explain how medications are taken and check whether the patient retains the information and insist on adherence.

• Show the particular techniques of administration of certain drugs (inhalation, injection, instillation of eye drops ...).

• Combating the phenomenon of self-medication.

• Teach the patient how to detect adverse effects, how to reduce the risk of their occurrence and explain what to do if they occur.

2. Integrate the patient into the therapeutic management of his disease:

❖ The pharmacist must explain to the patient the mechanisms of his disease, the action of the drugs, the expected benefits and the potential adverse effects. It is important to ensure that the patient has retained the information transmitted.

❖ It can also help the patient to participate in self-monitoring of amaladie (e.g. self-measurement of blood glucose by the glucometer or measurement of blood pressure by the electronic blood pressure monitor) or to detect warning signs of a 'major' adverse reaction.

Refrigerator products vaccination and injections

Refrigerator products, vaccination and injections

Refrigerator products:

These are heat-sensitive products that can deteriorate at room temperature.

These products are stored in the refrigerator at a temperature between 2°C and 8°C.

Vaccines:

› Pentavalent vaccine which includes diphtheria, tetanus, acellular pertussis, poliomyelitis vaccine and haemophilus type B (Pentaxim®/infranix)

› The pneumococcal vaccine (Prevenar®) designed for the prevention of pneumococcal disease.

› The combined live attenuated MMR vaccine (measles, mumps and rubella vaccine (Priorix®)

› Intradermal freeze-dried BCG vaccine which is indicated only at birth as soon as possible in a single dose.

› The hepatitis B vaccine

› Tetanus vaccine (Tetavax®)

Insulins:

We distinguish

› Rapid-acting insulins (Actrapid®)

› Ultra-fast insulin analogues: in pre-filled pen (Novorapid®)

› Insulins of intermediate action: (Insulatard®)

› Slow-acting insulin analogues (lantus,levemir®®)

› Rapid insulin analogues + Intermediate duration of action insulin (Novomix®)

› Rapid insulin + Intermediate duration of action insulin (Mixtard®)

Other products:

› Some eye drops (Xalacom®)

› Antibiotics (Rifocin ® ...)

Injections:

The practice of any injection is carried out only under medical prescription and any injection performed must be transcribed on the injection register issued by the CNOPT quoted and initialed by the pharmacist inspector. It should be noted:

> The date of the injection
> The name of the prescribing physician
> The numberm and first name of the patient
> The drug
> The mode of administration

Pharmacists are authorized to perform injections on medical prescription as well as pharmacy preparers under the responsibility of the pharmacist provided they hold an injection diploma.

Vaccination:

Vaccinations are one of the essential means of preventing infectious and viral diseases. They protect children and reduce the risk of epidemics. Some are mandatory, others are only recommended.

For each vaccine, respect the number of injections and do not neglect boosters

The pharmaceutical preparations

Officinal preparations and magistral preparations

1) Officinal preparations:

Definition:

'Compendial preparation' means any medicinal product prepared in a pharmacy, entered in the pharmacopoeia or national formulary and intended to be dispensed directly to patients supplied by that pharmacy.

Execution

› The preparation will be designated by the name it has in the National Formulary or in the Pharmacopoeia.

› Identify the formula of the preparation at the level of the booklet reserved for the preparations.

› Check the presence of raw materials and put them on the bench, otherwise order them

› Check the presence of the necessary equipment

› ��� the quantity of each plantto be sampled

› Use the electronic scale for weighing, for liquid forms use the specimen, pipette or dropper

› The preparation is carried out in accordance with the procedure indicated on the preparation sheet. Choosethe appropriate packaging.

› Write the preparation on the preparation book Label

› Pricing of preparation

› Check the stock of officinal preparations

Labelling:

Must be mentioned

› Surname, first name and address of the pharmacist.

› The full composition of the preparation or the name assigned to the medicinal product in the Pharmacopoeia or the National Formulary

› Dosage and instructions for use

Preparation	**INTERNAL channel (injectable, oral, nasal, sublingual, rectal, urethral and vaginal)**	**EXTERNAL (cutaneous, auricular...)**
Not containing poisonous substances or containing poisonous substances in <u>exempt</u> doses	**White** label	**White** label + **Non-red** back label **"external use"**
Containing poisonous substances in <u>non-exempt</u> doses	**White** label + **Red** back label **"Do not exceed the prescribed dose"**	**Red** label + **Red** back label **"Do not swallow"**

Examples of officinal preparations:

ü Aqueous eosine 2%

Formula:

Eosine..............................20g

Distilled water....................... QSP1000ml

Procedure:

› Weigh the eosin powder and place it in a glass beaker
› Dissolve in less than the total amount required
› Transfer to a 1000ml measuring cylinder
› Adjust up to 1000ml with distilled water
› Mix and let stand.
› Filter on a gas strip
› Divide into clean, well-dried glass vials

› Condition and label the preparation.

Labelling:

Preparation intended for the external route does not contain poisonous substances so it is a white label with a non-red counter label "external use"

Pricing :

Price of the quantity of eosin used, price of distilled water, and corresponding compensation.

Indication :

Diaper rash, umbilicus care, superficial burns

ü Alcohol 60 % v/v

Formula

95 percent ethanol V/V..............632 ml (1000*60/95)

Distilled water.............................. QSP1000ml

Procedure:

› Transfer to a 1000ml measuring cylinder632 ml of 95% ethanol

› Adjust up to 1000ml with distilled water

› Mix and let stand.

› Divide into clean, well-dried glass vials

› Condition and label the preparation.

Labelling:

Preparation intended for the external route does not contain poisonous substances so it is a white label with a non-red counter label "external use"

Pricing :

Price of the quantity of alcohol 95% used, price of distilled water, and the corresponding compensation.

2) Magistral preparations:

Definition:

Magistral preparation means any medicinal product prepared according to a medical prescription intended for a specific patient, extemporaneously in a pharmacy.

Examples of magistral preparations:

ü Preparation for external use

Formula

dexeryl®...................2 tubes

Uciderm more®.............. 5 tubes

Ownership of constituents

uciderm plus: fucidic acid, betamethasone[1] (Dermocorticoides with antibacterials[2])

dexeryl: glycerol, paraffin, petroleum jelly [3](Topicals with trophic or protective action[4])

Indication

Adjunctive treatment of shallow superficial burns

Procedure:

On a clean marble plaque

› Empty the continuous dermal cream of 2 tubes of dexeryl®

› Stir in uciderm plus® dermal cream by fraction and homogenize until a homogeneous preparation is obtained

› Packaging and labelling the preparation

› transcription on the authorising officer

---

1. https://www.med.tn/medicament/recherche/dci:ACIDE%20FUSIDIQUE,%20BETAMETHASONE%20(VALERATE)
2. https://www.med.tn/medicament/recherche/sc:Dermocorticoides%20avec%20antibacteriens
3. https://www.med.tn/medicament/recherche/dci:GLYCEROL,%20PARAFFINE,%20VASELINE
4. https://www.med.tn/medicament/recherche/sc:Topiques%20%C3%A0%20action%20trophique%20ou%20protectrice

Validation and dispensing of prescriptions

The Ordinance

The prescription is a legal entity that engages the responsibility of the prescriber and the dispensing pharmacist vis-à-vis the beneficiary patient.

The prescriber can be a doctor, dentist, midwife or veterinarian

Validation of the order

The validation of the medical prescription is an essential pharmaceutical act that must precede the dispensing of drugs. It is an act that aims to detect possible prescribing errors that can have various causes, which ensures patient safety.

The validation of the medical prescription is done in 2 main steps

Regulatory validation

The order must include

› Information on the prescriber: Surname, First name, contact details (address and telephone) possibly his CNAM code.

› Stamp and signature of the prescribing physician and the date of prescription.

› Patient information: Surname, First name, age, sex (and weight for children)

› Medicinal product(s): name(s), dosage form(s), dosage, dosage unit(s), route(s) of administration and duration of treatment

Pharmacological validation

Before dispensing medications, pharmacists must:

ü Take an interest in the patient:

Sex, age, weight, physiological status, history, medication history, self-medication

ü Be interested in medicines

› Identify the therapeutic objective

› Dosage study

› Establish a catching plan

› List adverse reactions

› Manage possible drug interactions

› Ensure the absence of contraindications to treatment

Enforcement of the order

After validation of the prescription and after ensuring the prescribed pharmaceutical form, it is necessary to

› estimate the number of units according to the duration of treatment.

› In the absence of mention of the duration, it will be necessary to issue the packaging most appropriate to the requirements of the prescription or to inquire with the prescriber.

› Check if the patient has social security coverage: National Health Insurance Fund (CNAM) or mutual STEG/SONED or another insurance.

If yes

› Identify the type of refund

› Check the validity of the care book and its compliance with the prescription

› Fill in the care book correctly

Dispensing medications by checking quantities, dosage and expiry date

possibly transcribe on the authorising officer

Information on the proper use of medicines

› Explain to the patient how to take the medication: frequency of intake, timing versus meal and duration of treatment

› Explain to the patient how to take medication (swallow, disperse...)

› Inform the patient about precautions for use and possible adverse effects.

› Educatesthe patient to medication adherence

› Draw the patient's attention to adverse effects and warning signs: for example signs of hypoglycaemia with oral antidiabetic agents

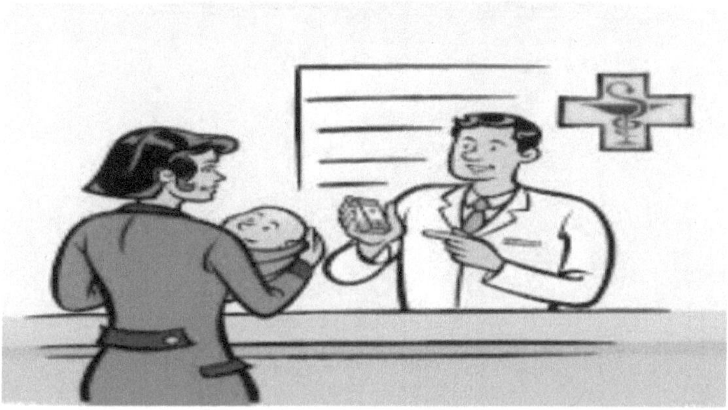

About the Author

"My name is Dr. Raafet.

'Dr.' refers to my last name, Dhkar, as well as my professional title as a doctor.

I hold a PhD in Pharmacy and I am passionate about sharing knowledge with others.

In order to provide easy access to knowledge, I publish my work on open platforms at an affordable price.

This allows students, researchers, and anyone interested to obtain valuable information without financial barriers.

I believe in the importance of granting individuals the opportunity to expand their understanding and contribute to the field of pharmacy."

www.ingramcontent.com/pod-product-compliance
Lightning Source LLC
LaVergne TN
LVHW090430210926
848480LV00002B/763